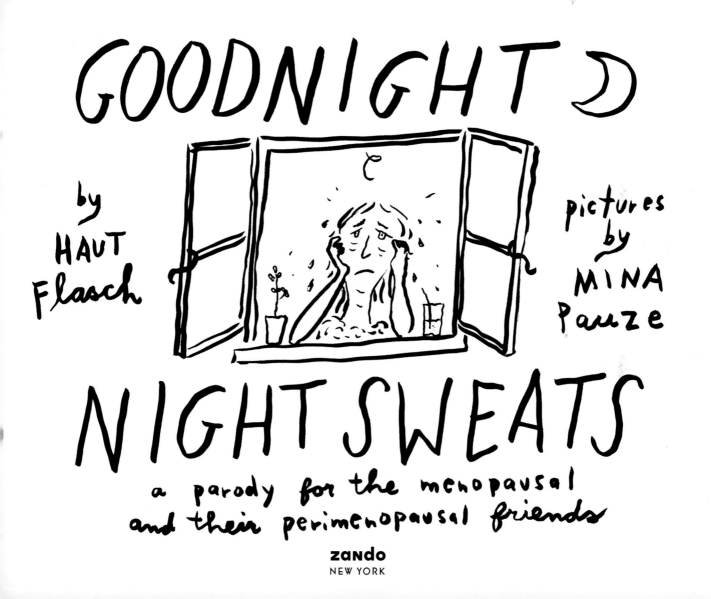

GOODNIGHT ☾

by **HAUT Flasch**

pictures by **MINA Pauze**

NIGHT SWEATS

a parody for the menopausal and their perimenopausal friends

zando
NEW YORK

For my sisters. All of them.—HF

To sweaty, mood-swinging women the world over.—MP

Thanks to our legendary agent Faye Bender; to the fabulous Molly Stern, Emily Bell, Evan Gaffney, and Maya Raiford-Cohen; and to everyone on the brilliant Zando team.

Text copyright © 2024 by Brenda Bowen
Illustrations copyright © 2024 by Jessie Hartland

Zando
zandoprojects.com

First Edition: March 2024

Cover illustration and design by Jessie Hartland
Text design by Pauline Neuwirth, Neuwirth & Associates, Inc.

The publisher does not have control over and is not responsible for author or other third-party websites (or their content).

978-1-63893-091-4 (Hardcover)
978-1-63893-092-1 (ebook)

1 3 5 7 9 10 8 6 4 2
Manufactured in China

In the hot, hot room

There was a creaky fan

And a swinging mood

And a picture of—

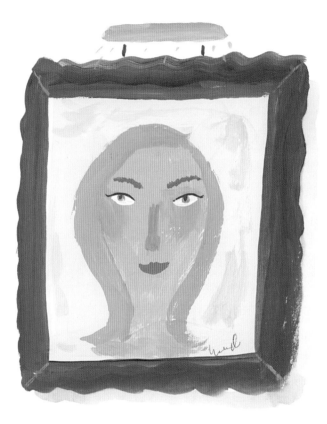

Me, while I was still in bloom

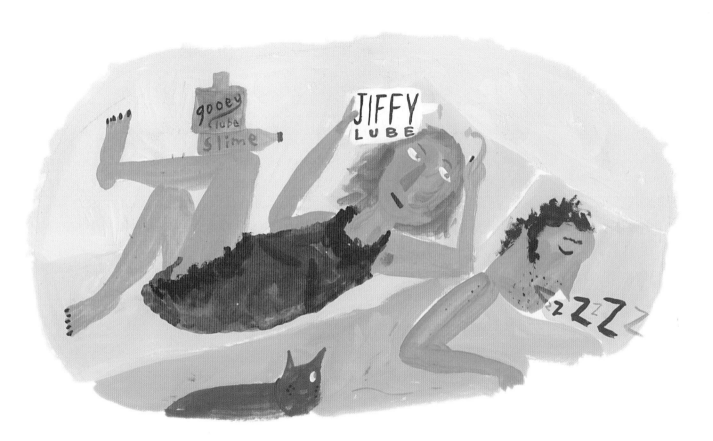

And there were two flat boobs

And three little lubes

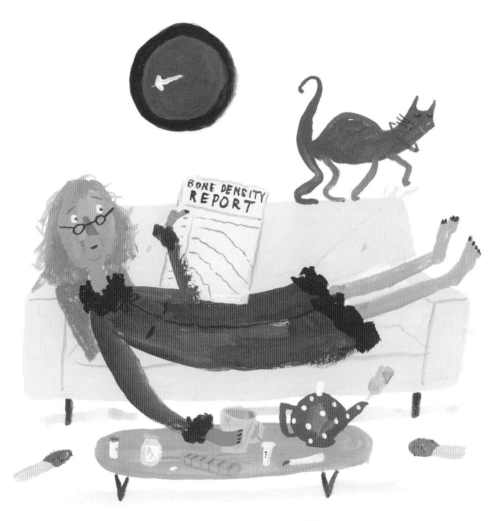

And bones like fine china

And a dry vagina

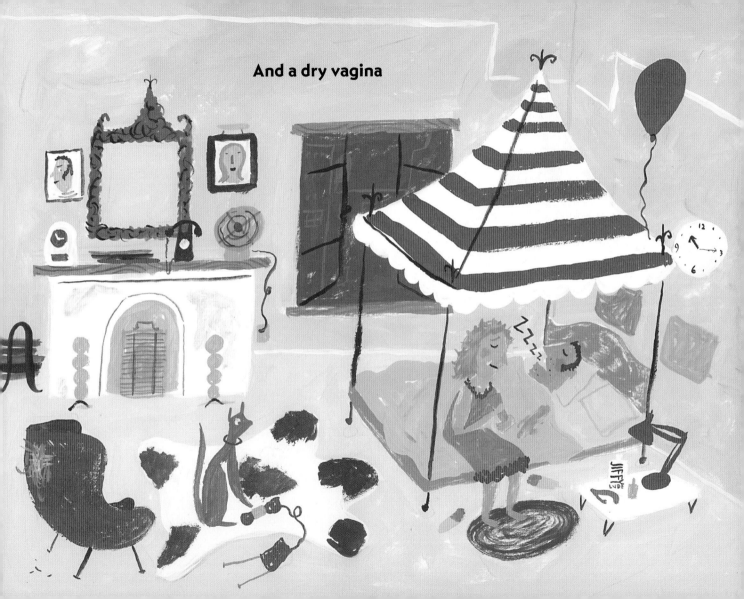

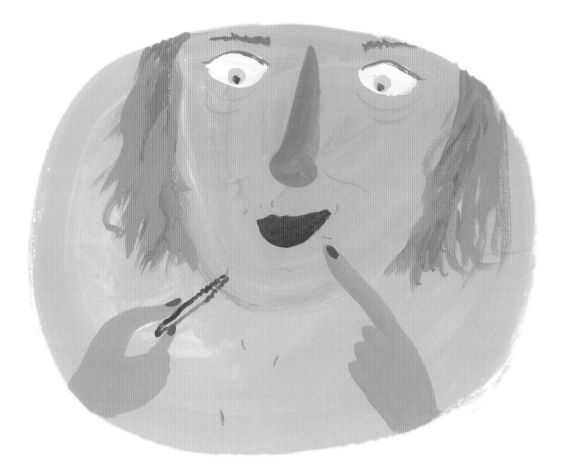

And a pair of tweezers

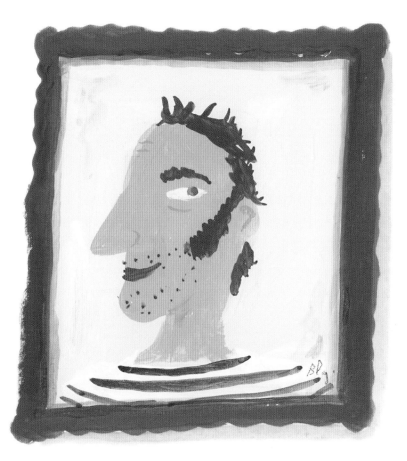

And a sweet old geezer

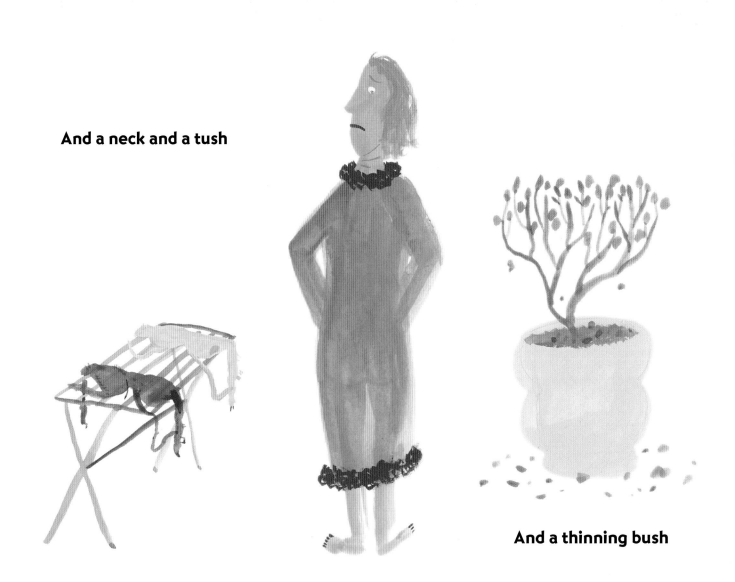

And a neck and a tush

And a thinning bush

And a middle-aged lady who's yelling,

"If I wake up drenched in sweat again tonight
I swear to God I will kill someone!"

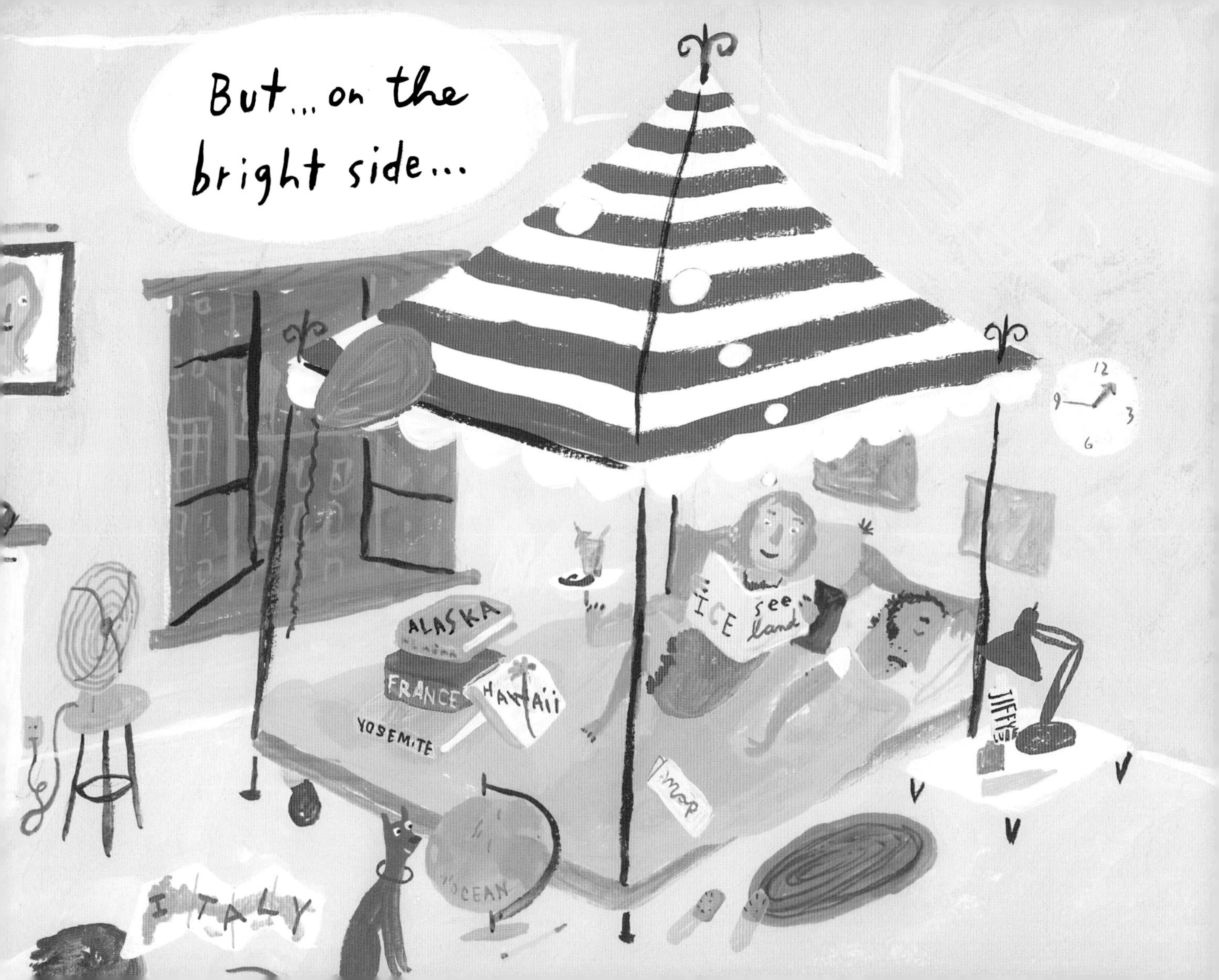

But... on the bright side...
ALASKA
FRANCE
HAWAii
YOSEMITE
ICE see land
Map
ITALY
OCEAN
JIFFY LUBE

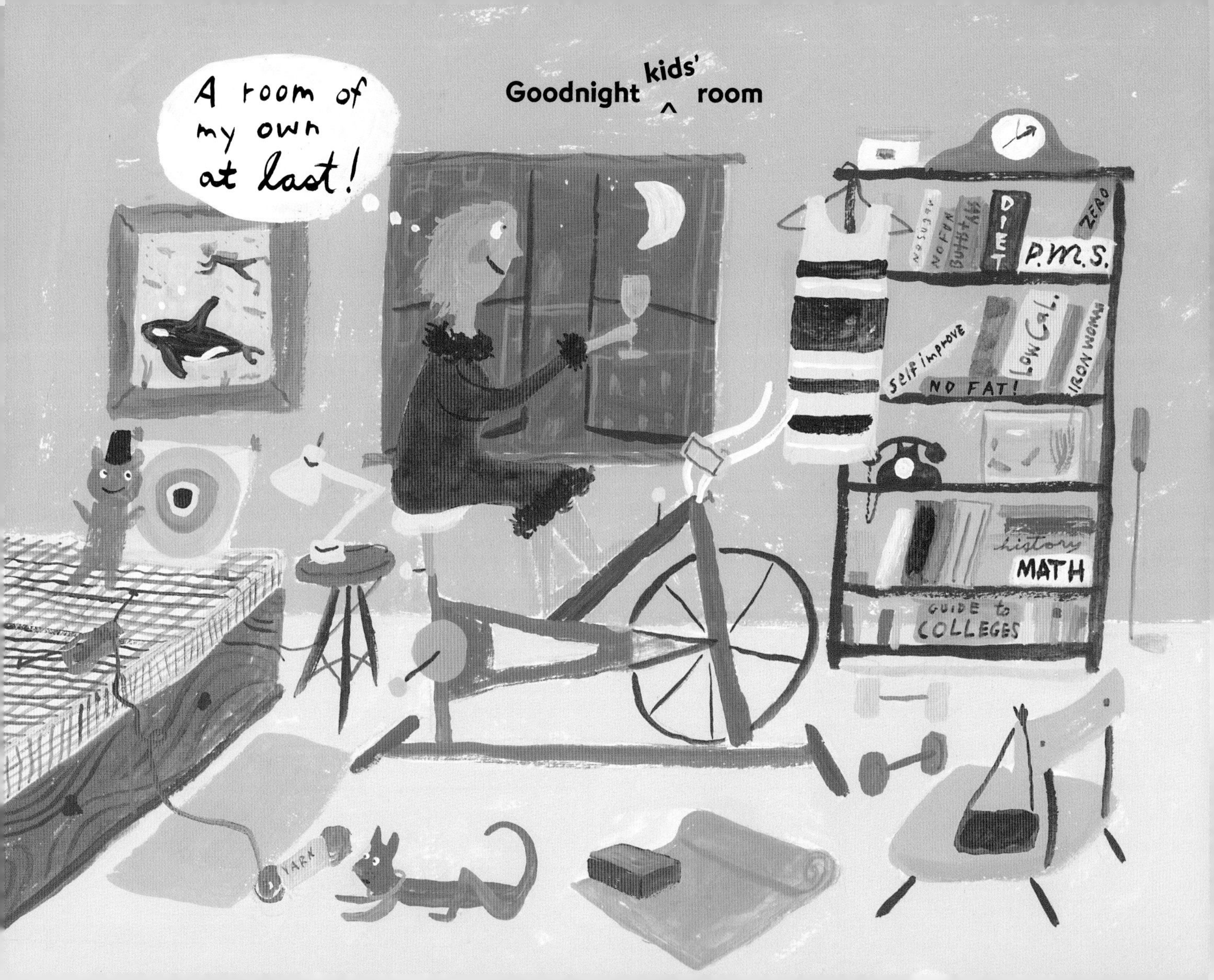
Goodnight kids' room
A room of my own at last!
DIET
ZERO
P.M.S.
Self improve
NO FAT!
Low Cal.
IRON WOMAN
history
MATH
GUIDE to COLLEGES

Goodnight gloom

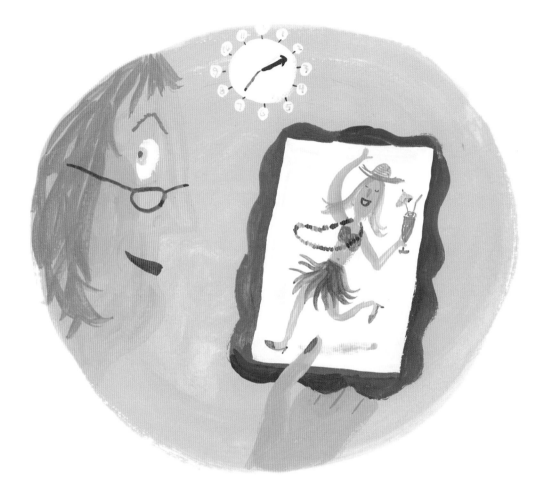

Goodnight me, while still in bloom

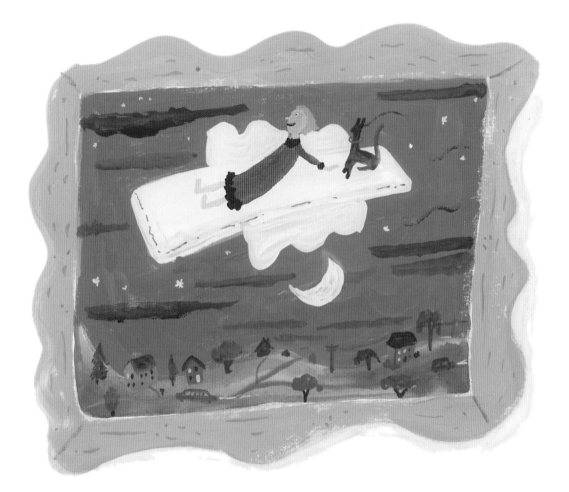

Goodnight wing'd pads and my dear old womb

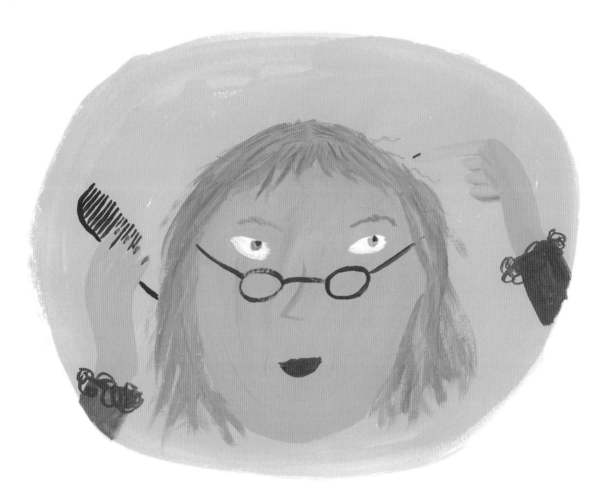

Goodnight dyeing the gray

And bizarre lingerie

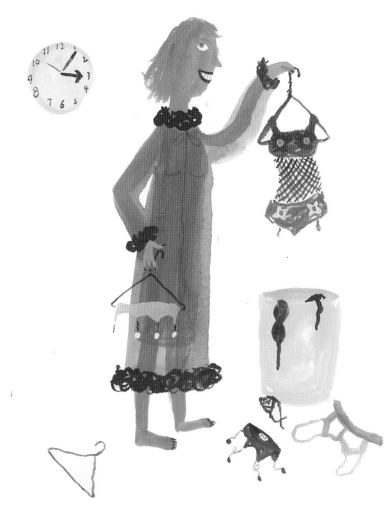

Goodnight cramps

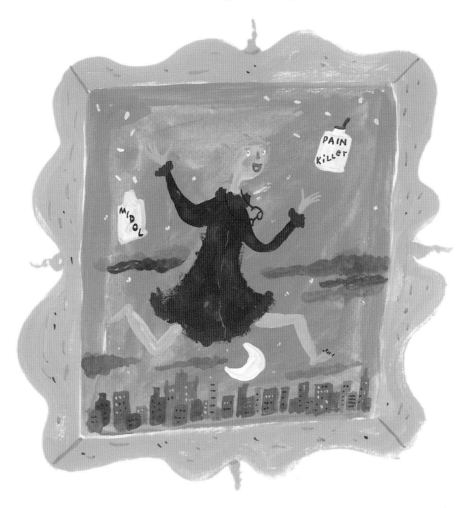

Goodnight stained pants

Goodnight bones like fine china

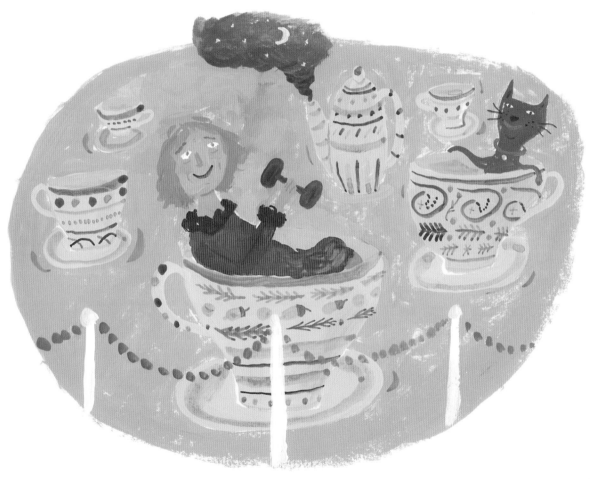

And *really* goodnight vagina!

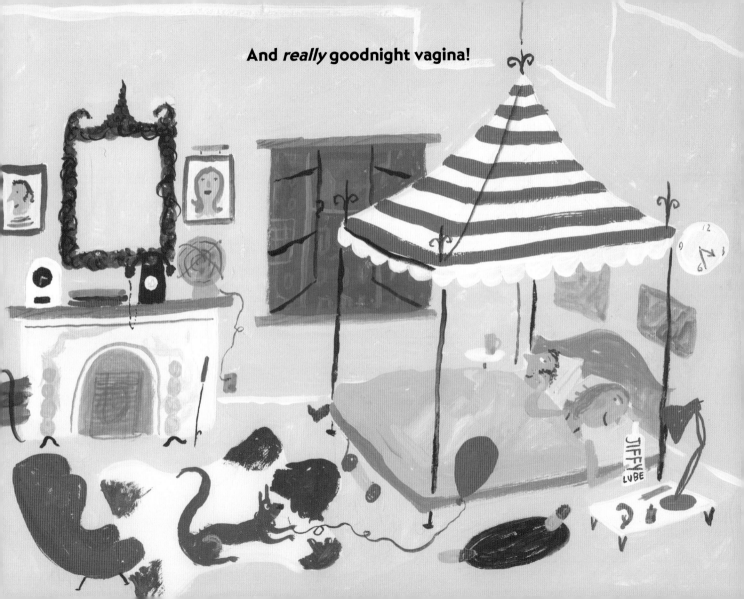

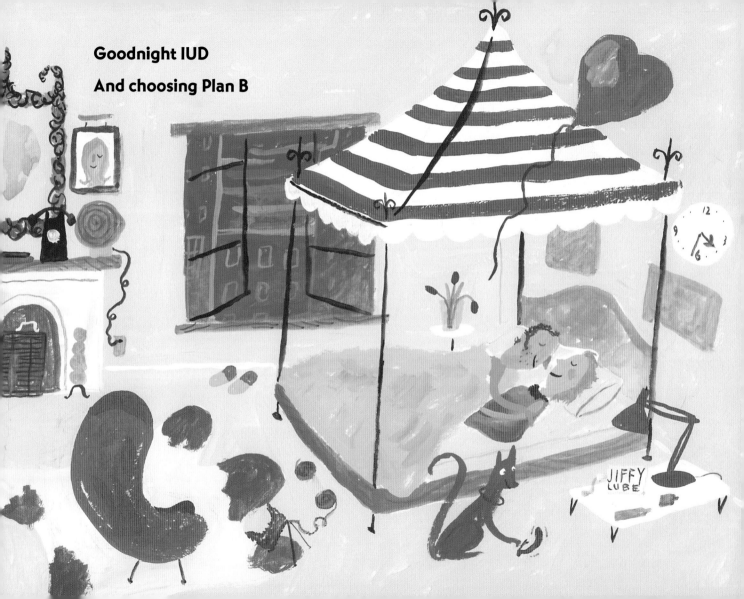

Goodnight IUD

And choosing Plan B

Goodnight period stress and PMS

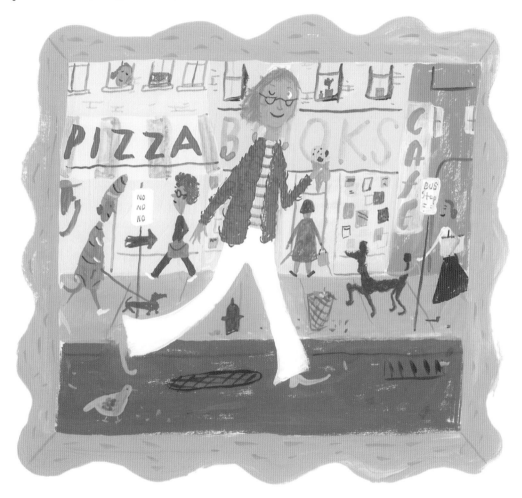

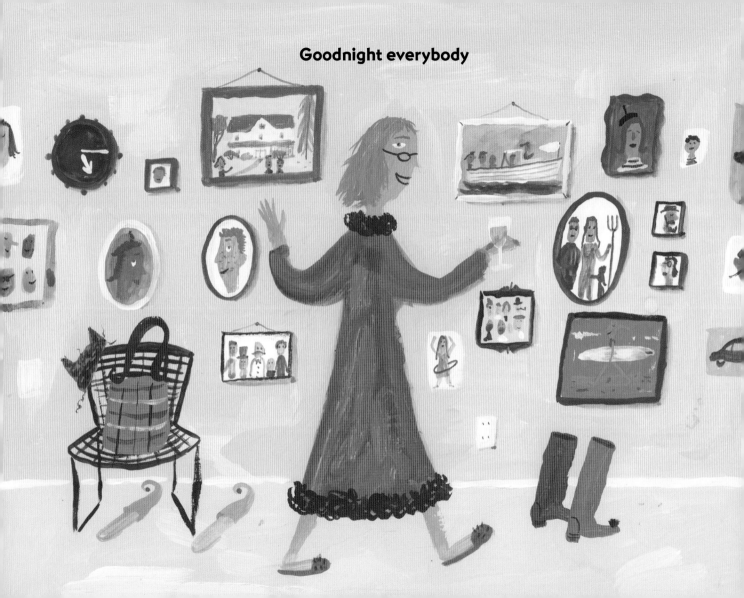

Goodnight everybody

And goodnight regrets

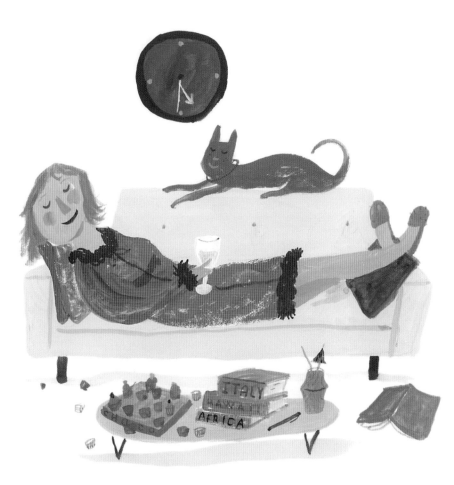

And goodnight to the hot-in-a-good-way lady calling,

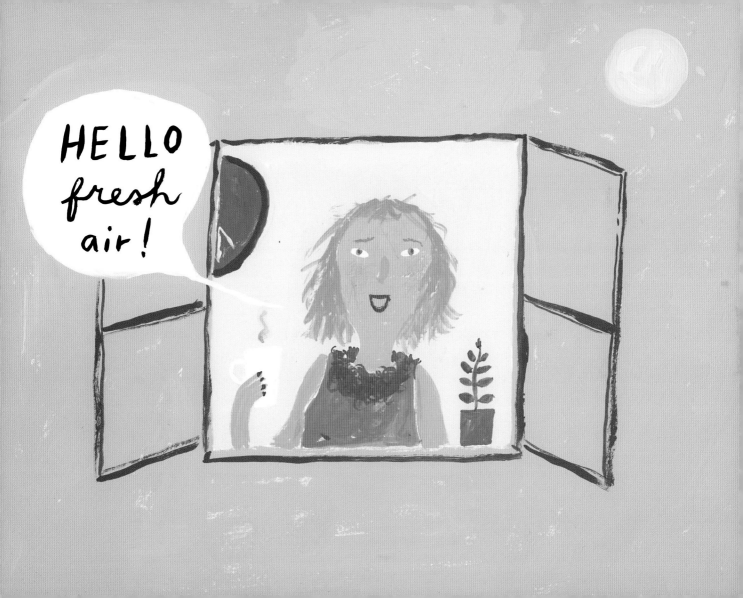

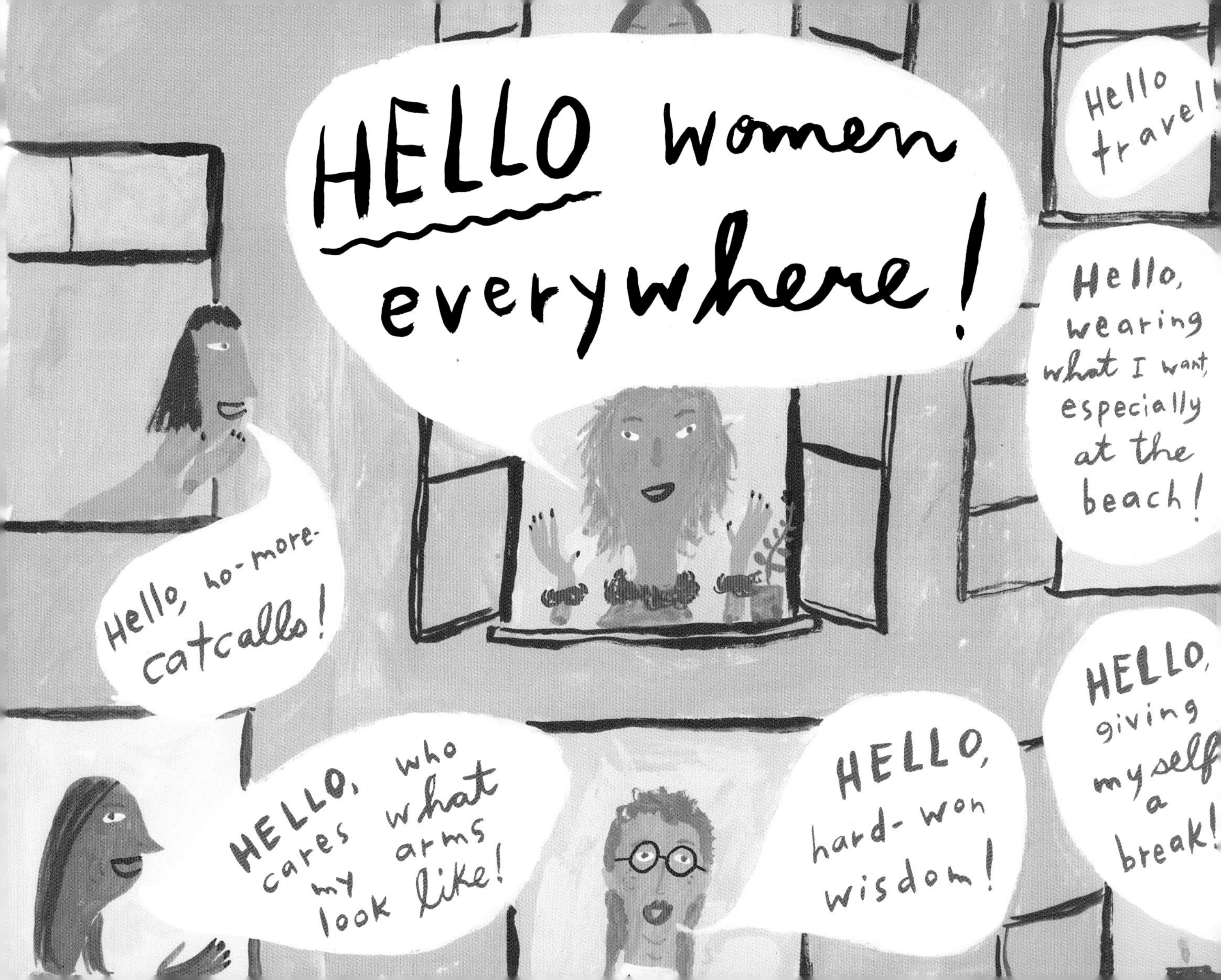
HELLO women everywhere!
Hello travel!
Hello, wearing what I want, especially at the beach!
Hello, no-more-catcalls!
HELLO, giving myself a break!
HELLO, who cares what my arms look like!
HELLO, hard-won wisdom!

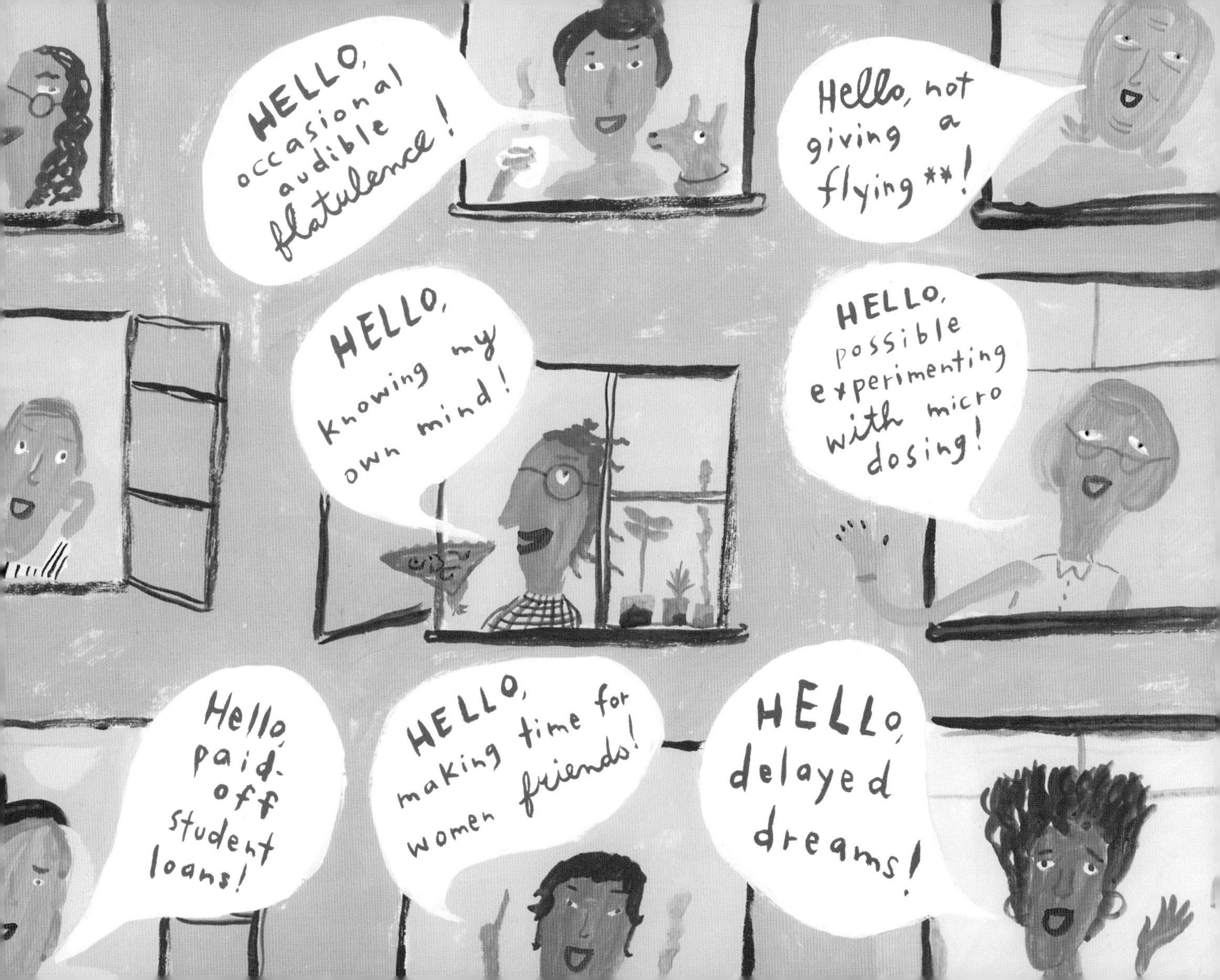

HELLO, occasional audible flatulence!
Hello, not giving a flying **!
HELLO, knowing my own mind!
HELLO, possible experimenting with micro dosing!
Hello, paid-off student loans!
HELLO, making time for women friends!
HELLO, delayed dreams!

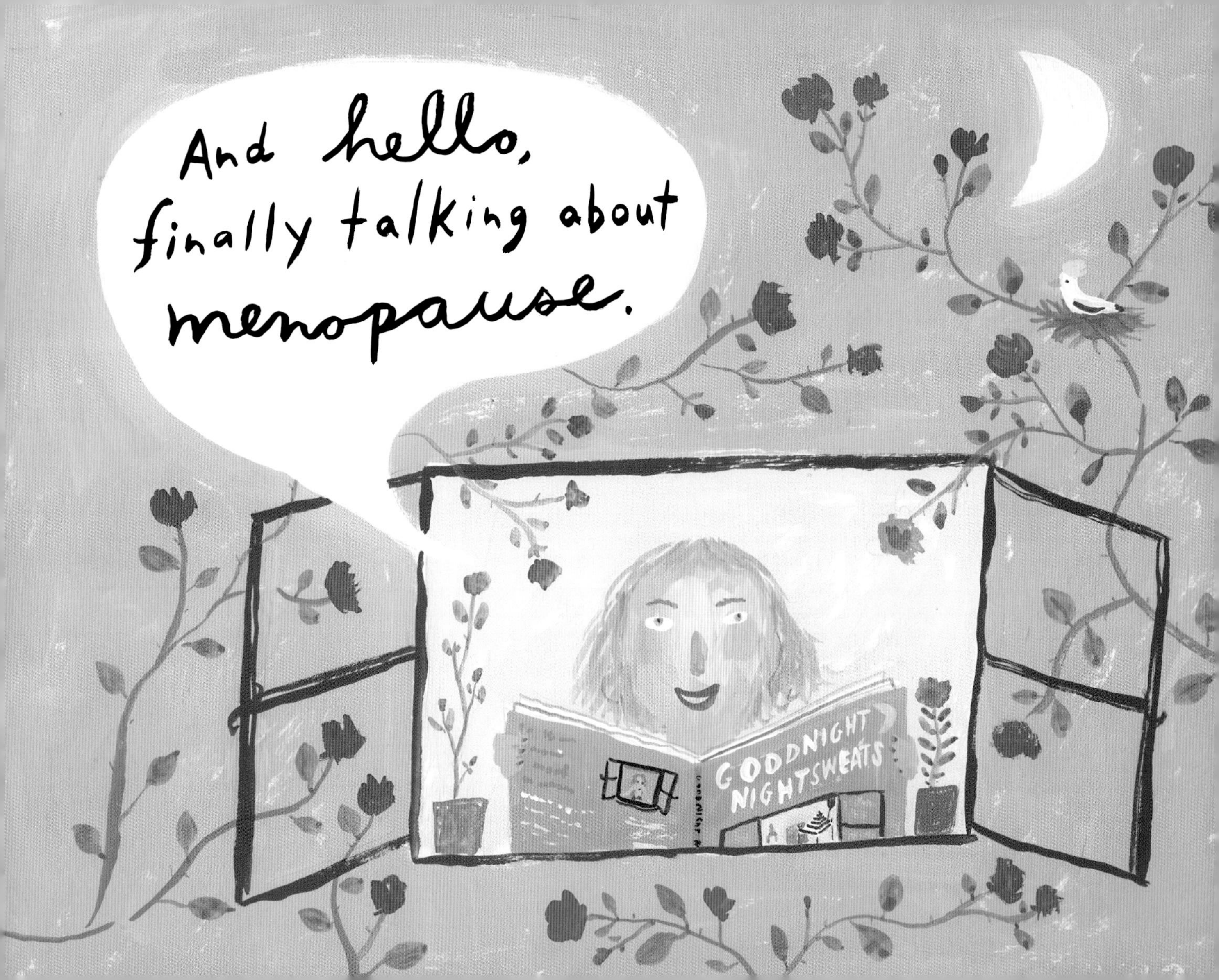
And hello,
finally talking about
menopause.
GOODNIGHT
NIGHTSWEATS